Food Is
Medicine

Nutritious and Delicious Recipes from my home shared with you

Jada Johnson

Food Is
Medicine

Nutritious and Delicious Recipes
from my home shared with you

Jada Johnson

Published by
Jada's R.O.A.R., LLC
Chesapeake, Virginia
2021

DISCLAIMER STATEMENT:

The information presented in this book is not intended to replace the recommendations and advice of your doctor. The presented information is not medical advice. The author is not responsible for injury or loss resulting from the use of the presented information. The presented information is based on the most current research available to the author at the time of publication. Mention of specific products does not constitute an endorsement.

Library of Congress Control Number: 2020925054
Johnson, Jada
ISBN: 978-1-7363005-0-3 (Paperback)
ISBN: 978-1-7363005-1-0 (eBook)
For bulk pricing ordering information, contact publisher at
jadasroar@gmail.com

Book Cover Design & Interior Layout: Scribe Freelance Book Designs Co.

Printed in the United States of America by
IngramSpark

Preface

Thank you, dad, for teaching me everything about the kitchen. You are my daily gourmet chef, and I love seeing you in action. I remember you showing me how to cut vegetables for the first time in elementary school, and I was so excited to learn! Your love for food and cooking is astronomical.

Thank you, mama, for teaching me the endless facts about nutrition. I love your passion and knowledge of this subject. You have taught me that there are hundreds of benefits to eating healthfully and staying strong.

Acknowledgements

"Food Is Medicine" was originally created for New Life Church NetCasters' Kitchen Ministry, located in Chesapeake Virginia, while completing my Girl Scout Gold Award. I saw the impact "Food Is Medicine" had on the participants of NetCasters' and wanted to share the information with many others.

- Thank you, Pastor Melvin, for introducing NetCasters' Kitchen Ministry to me.
- Thank you to my family and friends. All of you persuaded me to copyright and publish my book. Thank you for encouraging me to share my love for cooking and nutrition with everyone. The responses I receive as you try my recipes bring me so much enthusiasm.
- Recipe Testers: New Life NetCasters' Kitchen Ministry participants, Diabetes Prevention Program (DPP) learners and coaches at Sentara Virginia Beach General Hospital, registered dietitians, family and friends, and of course, my dad and mama.
- Editor: Nancy Gorry, RD, CDCES
- Proofreader: Susan De Abate, RN, MSN/ED, CDCES

This book is dedicated to my fellow Girl Scout sisters around the world. Always be respectfully heard, courageous in new adventures, and not let anyone or anything stand in the way of your dreams, just R.O.A.R....

Reach Out And Rule!

Introduction

I chose to write this book because I know the benefits of eating healthfully. Eating well affects behavior, well-being, and attitude. I learned this from my mama, her co-workers, and my teacher at school. If you do not eat healthfully, it can lead to nutrient deficiencies that cause poor growth, low energy, and illness. This book was written as a guide for people with prediabetes, diabetes, high blood pressure, high cholesterol, and heart disease. People without these conditions will also benefit. My goal for this book is to provide education while offering tasty dishes to inspire healthful selections.

I hope you enjoy these dishes from my home to yours! Please grow stronger, have more energy, and become resistant to illness and disease. Thank you for allowing me to provide this service to you.

Healthfully Yours,
Jada J.

Because of the Research...

The United States Department of Agriculture, the Academy of Nutrition and Dietetics, the American Diabetes Association, and the American Heart Association all suggest, a healthful eating pattern that includes fruits, vegetables, whole grains, low-fat and fat-free dairy, plant oils and lean protein foods. Together, these foods are full of nutrients that can help with improving and preventing diseases and maintaining good health, emphasizing:

Food Is Medicine

Frequently Used Ingredients and Things to Know

TBSP = tablespoon

tsp = teaspoon

Recommendations

Low sodium canned chicken broth or homemade prepared broths

- Low sodium foods are defined as having 140 mg of sodium or less per serving

> Each recipe serves 4, unless otherwise noted.

Milk: 1% low-fat or fat-free

- Low-fat foods are defined as having 3 grams of fat or less per serving

Plant Oils: olive and canola are best

- Plant oils have good effects on the blood fats (i.e., cholesterol and triglycerides)
- Other plant oils include corn, peanut, safflower, sesame, soybean, and sunflower
  - Try to avoid using lard, shortening, tropical oils (palm and coconut), and both stick butter and margarine. These have saturated fat and trans-fatty acids that can raise blood cholesterol.
  - Try to buy liquid, tub or spray butter and margarine. Remember, soft fats are more healthful than solid fats.

Vegetables

Fresh or frozen are best; however, if canned vegetables are preferred, make sure you drain and rinse the vegetables with water before cooking. Also, if possible, buy low sodium.

When using canned vegetables, the cook time in the recipes may differ from fresh.

Herbs

Basil, fresh	1 TBSP	=	1 tsp dried
Thyme, fresh	1 TBSP	=	1 tsp dried

Garlic, 1 medium sized clove = 1 tsp minced = ½ tsp garlic granules or garlic flakes = 1/8 tsp garlic powder.

Minced garlic has a strong flavor compared to the other options. Be careful not to burn the fresh garlic when cooking.

Salt and black pepper to taste   =   1/8 tsp or less of each

Salt-Free Seasonings

Use as much as your taste buds desire: garlic powder, granules or flakes, onion powder, dried onion, Italian seasoning, and herb mixtures. Please make sure the ingredient list on the label does not have "salt" listed.

INGREDIENTS: MARJORAM, THYME, ROSEMARY, SAVORY, SAGE, OREGANO, AND BASIL.

Added Sugars Include:

Table sugar, brown sugar, maple syrup and honey. The Guidelines for Healthy Americans recommend limited use of added sugars.

- Added sugars are also found in soda and other sugary drinks, candy, cookies, cakes, and pies.

Parmesan Cheese

Buy a wedge and shred it yourself! You will find an increase in flavor. Be cautious, some brands are higher in sodium than others. For a treat, try Parmigiano-Reggiano, also known as authentic parmesan cheese, the REAL DEAL.

Smoked Turkey Leg

Liquid smoke can be used in the place of a smoked turkey leg. Start with ½ tsp in the dish and adjust to taste.

Lemon or Lime

A lime can be used in the place of a lemon.

Simmer

Simmer means to turn the heat down and maintain a gentle bubbling. Some recipes will require this cooking technique.

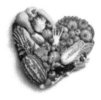

Table of Contents

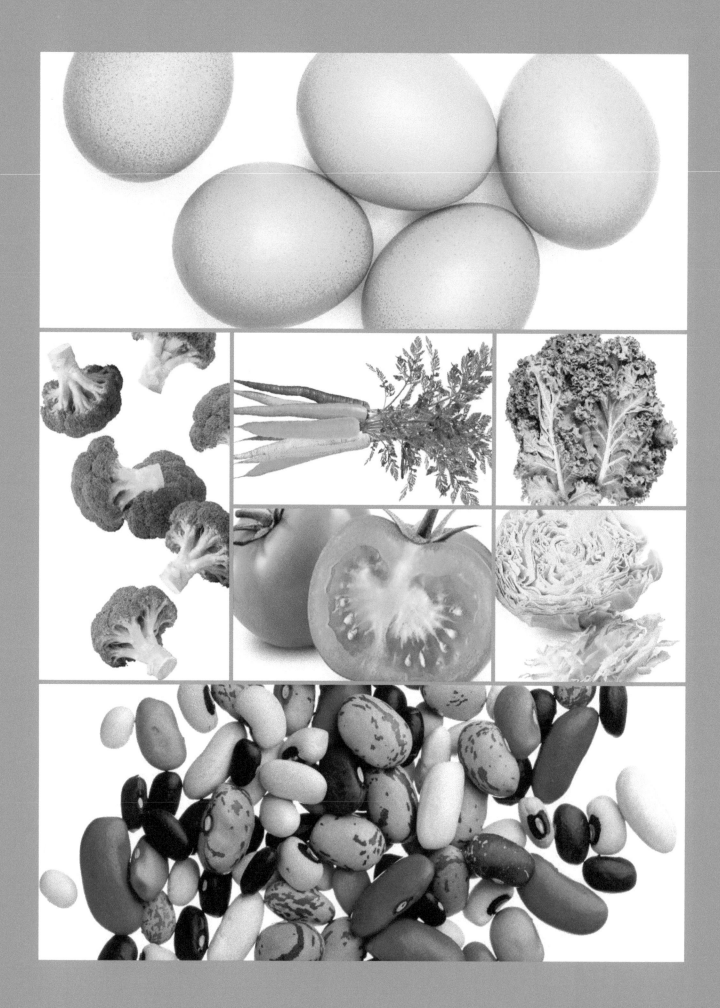

Why Vegetables?

Low calories
Low to moderate carbohydrates
No dietary cholesterol
No fat
Low to high fiber
High in vitamins and minerals
Low sodium
Low protein
Low to high phytonutrients and antioxidants
Help maintain good health
Wide variety of flavors and textures

Vegetables are rich in antioxidants. Antioxidants are substances that prevent damage to cells from free radicals. Too many free radicals in the body leads to diseases due to cell damage. Eating vegetables are good for heart health and may help reduce the risk of infections and some forms of cancer. Increase your antioxidant intake by eating more nuts, seeds, beans, fruits, and vegetables.

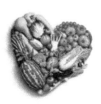

Why Beans?

- An excellent source of vegetable protein
- Cheapest protein on the market
- Lower LDL levels (bad cholesterol), making it good for the heart
- High in fiber, hence, promotes regular bowel movements
- Good source of antioxidants, potassium, iron, magnesium, and folate
- Helps control blood sugar, therefore, it's good for people who have diabetes

"What an easy, tasty way to get more beans in your diet! I swapped out the turkey leg for ham and let it cook itself all day in the slow cooker. I suggest pairing it with some rice and a veggie, and dinner is served!"

—April Rudat, MS Ed, RDN, LDN
(www.DietitianApril.com)

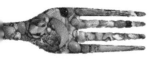

Mama's Beans

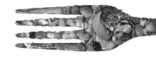

Ingredients

- 1 pound of your favorite dried beans (Navy, Pinto, Black Eyed Peas)
- 1 (14.5 ounce) can low sodium chicken broth
- 1 smoked turkey leg
- Salt and black pepper to taste
- 4 – 7 cups water

One hour after the start of cooking, check your beans. You may need to add 1-2 cups of water. Thereafter, every 30 – 45 mins, add an additional ½ - 1 cup of water, if needed.

Directions

1. Rinse beans in a colander, then set aside.
2. Bring the broth, turkey leg, salt, pepper, and 4 cups of water to a boil in a large pot. Add the beans, return to a boil.
3. Cover and simmer, until beans are tender. Stir occasionally.
4. Add warm water, if needed.
5. Cooking time will vary due to bean type.

Expect at least 2 hours. Once cooking is complete, remove the skin from turkey leg and chop the turkey meat into the beans.

Got Gas?

The carbohydrates in beans may cause short term digestive discomfort, also known as gas. Research shows that adding beans gradually to your eating pattern, at least once or twice a week, will help reduce the discomfort.

Crockpot It!

Adjust step 2 as follows: Add 3 cups water, broth, turkey leg, salt, pepper, and beans to crockpot. Cover and cook on low for about 10 hours.

Why Cabbage?

- High in vitamin C and vitamin K
- Good source of phytonutrients which may help prevent cancer, diabetes, and heart disease
- Good for the digestive system

Phytonutrients are natural compounds found in plant food. They act like antioxidants to help keep our cells healthy to prevent diseases.

Phytonutrients are found in a variety of fruits and vegetables.

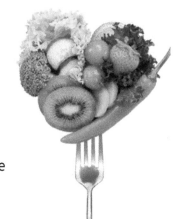

Grandma's Cabbage

Ingredients

- 1 head green cabbage, about 2 ½ -3 pounds (cut into strips)
- 1 (14.5 ounce) can low sodium chicken broth
- 1 smoked turkey leg
- 4 - 5 whole garlic cloves, minced (1 ½ - 2 TBSP)
- 1 1/2 TBSP olive oil
- ½ tsp black pepper
- Salt to taste
- 2 cups water

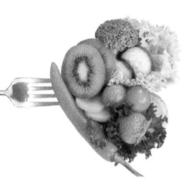

Prepare Cabbage:

Cut the cabbage in half. Place each half flat side down and cut down the middle. Cut off the stem (core) on each piece and discard. Place each quarter flat side down and cut into strips. Rinse cabbage in a colander.

Directions

1. Heat oil in a skillet on medium heat. Add the garlic and sauté for 2 to 3 minutes.
2. In a large pot bring to a boil the chicken broth, turkey leg, pepper, salt, and water. Add the garlic and any remaining oil in the skillet.
3. Add the cabbage and return to a boil.
4. Cover and simmer, stirring occasionally. Cook until tender, about 45 minutes to 1 hour.
5. Add warm water, if needed.
6. Once cooking is complete, remove the skin from the turkey leg, and chop the turkey meat into the cabbage.

Note: You can use this same recipe to cook 1 ¾ - 2 pounds of collard greens. Add 15 - 30 minutes to the cook time.

Why Tomatoes?

Tomatoes are a great source of potassium and lycopene. Potassium helps with fluid balance, muscle contractions, and nerve signals. Lycopene is a phytonutrient that helps protect cells from damage, keeping the heart healthy and helping to prevent cancer.

A tomato, just like other plant foods, does not have any dietary cholesterol because it is not an animal product. Also, tomatoes, along with most other fruits and vegetables, do not have any fat. How the vegetables are prepared may add fat.

Why Cucumbers?

Cucumbers contain vitamin K, folate, magnesium, and potassium. They have a high amount of water, which makes them delicious in a salad and refreshing sliced on a sandwich.

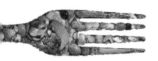

Magnesium is a mineral the body needs to contract and relax muscles, for example, moving your arms and legs. Some studies suggest a diet high in magnesium may help control blood glucose (sugar) levels. This is beneficial for people who have type 2 diabetes. Good sources of magnesium are dark green leafy vegetables, whole grains, beans, peas, lentils, and nuts.

Grape Tomato Pasta

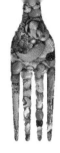

Ingredients

- 2 cups grape tomatoes
- 4 TBSP fresh basil, lightly chopped (or a little more than 1 TBSP dried)
- 1 TBSP olive oil
- 1 TBSP garlic, minced
- 2 cups penne pasta, cooked
- ¼ cup parmesan cheese

Directions

1. Cook the pasta according to package.
2. In the meantime, cut the tomatoes in half, lengthwise.
3. Heat oil in a pan on medium heat. Add the garlic and sauté for 2-3 minutes. Add the tomatoes and sauté until soft.
4. Add the basil.
5. Drain the pasta and mix with tomatoes while pasta is hot.
6. Serve and top it off with parmesan cheese.

> Lycopene is found in tomatoes. The body absorbs more lycopene when tomatoes are cooked, especially if cooked with oil.

Grape and Cherry Tomatoes, what's the difference?

> Grape tomatoes have thick skin, sweet taste, and an oblong shape like a grape.
>
> Cherry tomatoes have thin skin, much sweeter than grape tomatoes, round like a cherry and very juicy.

Herb Tomato and Cucumber Medley

Ingredients

- 2 cups cherry tomatoes, cut in half
- 1 cucumber (my favorite, English cucumbers)
- ½ medium red onion, thinly sliced then cut in half
- 2 TBSP olive oil
- 2 TBSP red wine vinegar
- 2 TBSP fresh parsley, lightly chopped (2 tsp dried)
- 4 TBSP fresh basil, lightly chopped (or a little more than 1 TBSP dried)
- Salt and black pepper to taste
- 1/3 cup feta cheese, optional

Note: You can use grape tomatoes or 2 of your favorite medium sized tomatoes cut into bite size pieces in the place of the cherry tomatoes.

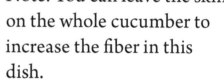

Directions

1. Peel skin off one half of the cucumber then thinly slice both halves.
2. Cut the cucumber slices in half.
3. Combine the tomatoes, cucumbers, and onions in a medium sized bowl.
4. Lightly season with salt and pepper.
5. In a small bowl, whisk the oil and red wine vinegar. Pour the dressing over the tomatoes, onions, and cucumbers, and gently stir.

Note: You can leave the skin on the whole cucumber to increase the fiber in this dish.

6. Add the herbs and gently stir. Cover and refrigerate for a couple of hours.
7. Before serving, sprinkle with feta cheese.

Honey Glazed Carrots

Ingredients

- 1-pound carrots, peeled and sliced into sticks
- 1 1/2 TBSP margarine
- 1 TBSP + 2 tsp honey
- 1 tsp dried rosemary
- ½ tsp garlic powder
- Salt to taste

Directions

1. Preheat the oven to 400 degrees.
2. In a saucepan, melt the margarine on low heat. Add the honey, rosemary, garlic, and salt.
3. Add the carrots to the mixture and coat well.
4. Pour carrots onto the baking sheet in a single layer.
5. Bake until caramelized and glazed, about 25 – 30 minutes.

Note: You can replace whole carrots with a 16-ounce bag of baby carrots. If desired, cut carrots in half lengthwise.

For easy clean-up, cover baking sheet with aluminum foil or parchment paper.

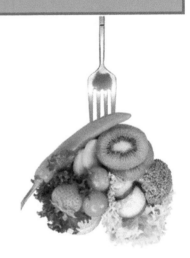

Carrots contain beta-carotene which can help lower the risk of cancer and heart disease. The body changes beta-carotene into vitamin A. Vitamin A helps keep the skin and eyes healthy and the immune system strong.

Vegetable Pasta

Ingredients

- 1 cup cooked pasta, drained
- 1 cup fresh broccoli, washed and cut into bite size florets
- 1 cup cherry tomatoes cut in half
- 1/2 cup shredded carrot

For the Dressing

- ½ cup white wine vinegar
- 2 TBSP olive oil
- 2 TBSP water
- 2 tsp dried basil leaves
- 2 tsp dried oregano leaves
- 2 tsp garlic powder
- Black pepper to taste

> Broccoli is a good source of vitamin C, folate, and phytonutrients. Eat it raw or steam, stir-fry, sauté, or microwave less than one minute to retain the nutrients.

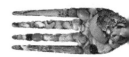

Directions

1. Mix in a small bowl the vinegar, oil, water, basil, oregano, garlic, and pepper, set aside.
2. Combine pasta, broccoli, tomatoes, and carrots in a large bowl. Pour dressing over the pasta mixture. Toss until evenly coated.
3. Cover and refrigerate for at least 4 hours to blend flavors.

Note: Consider preparing this dish in the morning to allow it to marinate throughout the day to serve with dinner. The longer it is in the refrigerator, the better it will taste!

Instead of making the dressing, you could use your favorite Italian or vinaigrette dressing. Be cautious, some brands are higher in sodium than others.

Why Eggs?

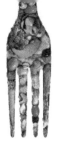

- Moderate in calories
- High in protein
- Low in fat
- High in cholesterol
- Low in sodium

Eggs do not have fiber. Adding chopped vegetables during cooking will add fiber.

Eggs are rich in choline, lutein, and vitamin D, all of which are found in the yolk of the egg. Choline helps with memory and learning. Lutein helps keep the eyes healthy.

Vitamin D helps absorb calcium into the body. Eggs contain a little calcium. Calcium prevents the bones from being porous (with holes). Porous bones break easily. Vitamin D also helps keep the immune system strong. Additional sources of vitamin D are sunlight, fatty fish, and fortified dairy foods, juices, and cereals.

> The best sources of calcium are milk, cheese, and yogurt.

Q: What's the difference between white and brown eggs?

A: the hen

Red-feathered hens lay brown eggs, and white-feathered hens lay white eggs. Red-feathered hens are often bigger, so they eat more. This is why brown eggs cost a little more in the store. The nutrition makeup is the same.

Spinach Quiche

Ingredients

- 1 deep dish frozen or homemade pie crust
- 1 (10oz) box frozen spinach
- 3 eggs, beaten
- 1 cup milk
- ½ cup green onion, sliced
- 1 cup chopped cooked chicken (seasoned and grilled is my favorite)
- 1 cup cheddar cheese
- ½ cup parmesan cheese
- 1 TBSP flour
- Dash nutmeg
- Salt and black pepper to taste

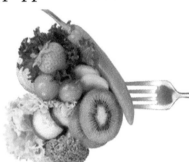

Directions

1. Randomly prick holes in frozen pie crust with fork (about 15 pricks). Don't forget the sides. Line the shell with foil. Bake in the oven at 450 degrees for 5 minutes. Remove foil slowly (to make sure no crust got on the foil) and bake an additional 6 - 7 minutes more or until pastry is nearly done. Remove from oven.
2. Reduce oven temperature to 325 degrees.
3. Meanwhile, thaw the spinach in the microwave or stove top: bring 1 cup water in a pot to a boil. Add the spinach. Turn down the heat and break the spinach up until separated. Drain well in a colander and pat dry with paper towels. Season with salt and pepper.
4. In a small bowl, mix the cheeses, and toss with the flour. Set aside.
5. In another bowl, stir the eggs, milk, onions, chicken, spinach, nutmeg, salt, and pepper. Add cheese and mix well.
6. Pour all into the pie crust.
7. Bake for 45 - 50 minutes or until a knife inserted near the center comes out clean.

Change it up!

Instead of using 3 whole eggs try...
2 whole eggs plus 2 egg whites.

Instead of cheddar and parmesan try 1 ½ cup mix of your
favorite cheeses, for example...
1 cup Monterey Jack + ½ cup cheddar OR
¾ cup swiss + ¾ cup mozzarella

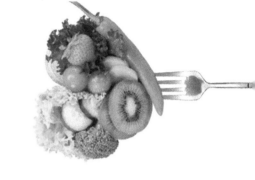

Instead of frozen spinach, use fresh spinach.
10oz frozen is about 3 cups packed fresh spinach. You can
add it raw or cook it down 2 - 3 minutes in a little water.
Make sure you drain and pat dry on paper towel. Season
with salt and black pepper.

Instead of chicken try...
1 cup cooked, seasoned chopped lean protein of your choice.

OR

1 cup mushrooms: Heat 1 tsp olive oil in a pan on medium heat. Add 1 tsp minced
garlic and sauté about 2-3 minutes. Add the mushrooms, then salt and pepper. Sauté
on medium heat for about 6 -7 minutes until there is no water at the bottom of the
pan. Pat dry on a paper towel.

Note: To prevent a soggy quiche, get rid of the moisture in your vegetables.
Mushrooms, when cooked, release a lot of liquid. Cooking your mushrooms
beforehand will reduce the moisture in them.

Why Mushrooms?

Mushrooms are a good source of the mineral selenium, an antioxidant that may help reduce the risk of some diseases. Riboflavin is a B vitamin, also found in mushrooms. The body uses B vitamins to break down fat and protein and to convert carbohydrates into glucose to produce energy for the cells.

Sauted Mushrooms

- 2 cups mushrooms (my favorite, baby bella)
- 1 TBSP olive oil
- 5 cloves garlic, minced (2 TBSP)
- 1 TBSP dried thyme
- Salt and pepper to taste

Directions

1. In a medium sized pan, add the oil on medium heat.
2. Add the garlic and sauté for 2 – 3 minutes.
3. Add the mushrooms, thyme, salt, and pepper. Cook until tender, about 4 – 6 minutes. Serve on top of rice or potatoes.

> These are perfect with "Cauliflower Mashed Potatoes" pg. 17, "Homemade Tomato Sauce" pg. 27 and on top of your "Mushroomed Burger" pg. 60.

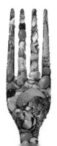

Cauliflower Mashed Potatoes

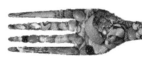

Ingredients

- 2 heads cauliflower, cut into florets and washed
- 1 TBSP olive oil
- 1 tsp margarine
- 2 TBSP garlic, minced
- ¼ cup parmesan cheese
- Salt and black pepper to taste

Cauliflower is a good source of vitamin C. Vitamin C helps the body absorb iron. Iron is needed to carry oxygen throughout the body. If your iron is low, you may feel tired often.

Directions

1. In a large pot, add enough water to cover the cauliflower, bring to a boil.
2. Add the cauliflower and cook until fork tender, about 15 to 20 minutes.
3. Meanwhile, heat olive oil in skillet over medium heat.
4. Stir in the garlic and sauté 2-3 minutes. Remove from heat.
5. Drain cauliflower well. Remove as much water as possible.
6. Mash with a potato masher or fork.
7. In a large bowl, mix the mashed cauliflower, garlic, parmesan cheese, and margarine.
8. Season with salt and pepper.

Cauliflower provides phytonutrients that can help block cancer cell growth. It also contains fiber to help keep you feeling full after eating a meal, and choline that is needed for learning and memory.

> "I cannot believe this is cauliflower and not mashed potatoes."
> —NetCasters' Kitchen Ministry participants and DPP learners

Why Zucchini?

Zucchini is a type of squash. Zucchini has potassium and vitamin C. Vitamin C is a water-soluble vitamin that is important for boosting immunity, repairing cells, and slowing down the aging process.

Why Green beans?

Potassium is the main mineral in green beans. Eating foods high in potassium may help control blood pressure. Green beans also have some vitamin C.

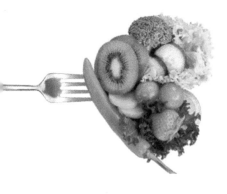

Mixed Vegetables

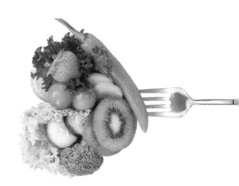

Ingredients

- 2 cups green beans, cut into 1-inch pieces
- 1 small onion, chopped
- 1 TBSP + 2 tsp olive oil
- 2 small zucchinis, cut into 1/4-inch slices
- 3 bacon strips, center cut, cooked, and crumbled (smoked turkey meat could work too)
- Salt and black pepper to taste
- 1 cup water

Directions

1. In a pot, bring the water to a boil. Add the green beans. Return to a boil and cook, uncovered, for 8-10 minutes or until the beans are tender. Drain.
2. Meanwhile, in a large skillet, on medium heat, sauté the onion in 1 TBSP oil for 3 minutes or until tender. Add the remaining oil and zucchini. Sauté for 4 minutes or until vegetables are tender. Stir in the bacon, green beans, salt, and pepper. Heat through.

> Note: Bacon, bologna, salami, and hot dogs are high in sodium and fat. Try not to eat these foods all the time.

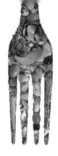

Parmesan Green Beans

Ingredients

- 2 cups green beans
- 1 - 1 ½ TBSP olive oil
- ½ tsp onion powder
- 1 tsp garlic powder
- ¼ tsp black pepper
- Salt to taste
- ¼ cup parmesan cheese

Directions

1. Preheat the oven to 425 degrees.
2. In a large bowl, combine the oil, onion powder, garlic powder, pepper, and salt.
3. Add the green beans and toss. Spread beans evenly on a baking sheet.
4. Bake 15 minutes, stir, and cook another 10 – 15 minutes.
5. Sprinkle beans with the parmesan cheese and return to the oven for 1 – 2 minutes (or until cheese is melted).

Note: One pound of Brussel sprouts, cauliflower florets, or broccoli florets in place of the green beans, will also work well with this recipe. Wash and prepare the vegetables.

- For the Brussel sprouts, slice off the ends and cut in half. Fresh squeezed lemon juice sprinkled evenly on sprouts adds a nice flavor. Squeeze lemon juice at the same time parmesan cheese is added.

> Brussel sprouts are related to cabbage, broccoli, cauliflower, and kale. Brussel sprouts are rich in vitamin K, which is good for blood clotting. This vegetable is also a good source of beta-carotene, lutein, and the antioxidant vitamin C. High in fiber, Brussel sprouts support the digestive system.

Three Bean Salad

Ingredients

- 1 (15 ounce) can black beans, drained and rinsed
- 1 (15 ounce) can pinto beans, drained and rinsed
- 1 (15 ounce) can cannellini beans, drained and rinsed
- 1 (12 ounce) can corn, drained and rinsed
- ¾ cup celery, chopped
- 1 cup onion, chopped
- ¾ cup sweet pepper (all colors), chopped
- ½ cup apple cider vinegar
- ¼ cup canola or olive oil
- ¼ cup sugar

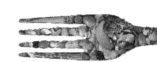

Directions

1. Mix the beans and vegetables in a large bowl and set aside.
2. In a pot, bring to a boil the oil, sugar, and vinegar. Simmer for 2 minutes, then pour over the beans and vegetables. Stir well.
3. Keep in the refrigerator for at least 4 hours, stirring occasionally.

Consider preparing this dish in the morning to allow it to marinate throughout the day. Serve with baked tortilla chips as an appetizer or as a side at a meal. Serves 6.

> Try with "Homemade Pita Chips" pg. 51.

Note: Use low sodium canned beans and corn if available. Replace beans in the recipe with your favorite beans. Garbanzo and red kidney beans work well in this dish too.

Creamed Spinach and Mushrooms

Ingredients

- 1 TBSP + 1 tsp olive oil
- 1/3 cup onions, chopped
- 1 TBSP garlic, minced
- 1 cup mushrooms
- 4 cups baby spinach, fresh
- ¾ cup milk
- 1 TBSP all-purpose flour
- Salt and black pepper to taste
- 1 dash of nutmeg
- 1/3 cup non-fat Greek yogurt
- ¼ cup parmesan cheese, optional

Spinach is an excellent source of iron, vitamin K, and vitamin A. Spinach is also a good source of vitamin C, magnesium, and potassium.

Directions

1. In a medium sized pan, heat 1 TBSP oil on medium heat. Add onions and garlic and sauté for 1 minute. Add the mushrooms and sauté for an additional 5 – 6 minutes. Place in a bowl and set aside.
2. Using the same pan, add 1 tsp of oil and the spinach. Cook for one minute, or until the spinach is wilted.
3. Remove spinach from pan and add to the mushroom mixture. Clean pan.
4. In another bowl, mix the milk and flour, then add it with the salt, pepper, and nutmeg to your pan on low heat stirring constantly. Cook for 3 minutes or until thick. Add Greek yogurt and stir until mixture is smooth.
5. Add the mushrooms, spinach, garlic, and onions to the milk mixture. Toss gently to coat. Once plated, sprinkle parmesan cheese on top.

Note: Kale in the place of the spinach tastes good in this recipe, too.

Lemony Kale Spaghetti

Ingredients

- 1 bunch curly kale, washed and dried
- 3 TBSP olive oil
- 2-3 TBSP freshly squeezed lemon juice (1 medium sized lemon)
- 2–3 TBSP Italian seasoning, salt free
- Black pepper to taste
- 2 cups spaghetti pasta, cooked
- ¼ cup parmesan cheese

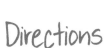

Directions

1. Remove the stems from the kale and cut into thin strips.
2. Place the kale in a bowl. Add the oil, lemon juice, Italian seasoning, and pepper, toss and set aside to marinate.
3. While the kale is marinating, cook the spaghetti according to package. Before draining, keep one cup of the cooking water. Add the pasta to the bowl with the kale and toss together well. Add ½ cup of the pasta water to moisten the dish. If needed, add additional ½ cup.
4. Add the cheese and toss.

This is one of my favorite side dishes. Kale tastes great when you add it to homemade soups, too.

> Kale is rich in vitamin K, vitamin A, and the antioxidant vitamin C which can help prevent cancer. Kale is also a good source of phytonutrients beta-carotene and lutein.

Why Collard Greens?

Collard greens have folate, also known as vitamin B-9. Folate is important for brain development and function. Collards are a good source of vitamin A, vitamin K, calcium, and phytonutrients, lutein, and beta-carotene. Research has shown both compounds, lutein and beta-carotene may decrease the risk of cancer and heart disease. Lutein is also linked to eye health. Collard greens are also rich in magnesium and potassium.

"My nephew Roni is an awesome cook, and to know he has instilled the love of cooking into his daughter, is not a surprise. His collard greens will take you to a happy place."

—Aunt Faye

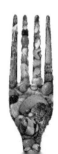

Daddy's Crunchy Collards

Ingredients

- 1 ¾ - 2 pounds collard greens
- 2 TBSP olive oil
- 1 cup smoked turkey leg meat, chopped
- 3 TBSP garlic, minced
- 2 (14.5 ounce) cans low sodium chicken broth

- ¼ cup white vinegar
- ½ + ½ cup water
- ½ tsp salt
- 1 tsp black pepper
- 2 TBSP maple syrup
- 1 tsp cayenne pepper, optional

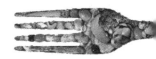

Directions

1. Wash the greens in cold water until free of dirt. Remove the thick stems from the greens by slicing along the side of the stem with a knife (or use your hands to remove the greens from the stem).
2. Stack several greens on top of each other and roll them up like a cigar. Slice the roll in 1-inch sections. Repeat with all the greens. Place greens in a large bowl, cover with paper towels, and set in the refrigerator until needed.
3. In a medium sized bowl, add the turkey meat and garlic. Mix well.
4. Heat the oil in a pan on medium heat. Add the turkey and garlic mixture and fry for 4 – 6 minutes. Stir occasionally.
5. In a large pot, add the chicken broth, vinegar, and ½ cup of water. Bring to a boil then add the turkey mixture.
6. Stir in the salt and pepper. Allow the mixture to simmer for 2 – 4 minutes, then add the greens. Stir well.
7. Cover and cook on medium high heat for 30 minutes. Check the greens in 15 minutes and add water, if needed.
8. Add the maple syrup and cayenne pepper, if using. Add ½ cup of water, toss the greens around and bring to a boil.
9. Cover and simmer for 10 – 15 minutes, tossing occasionally. Serves 4 – 6.

I'm proud to say, my dad won a contest making these collards.

Why Lycopene?

Lycopene is a phytonutrient that helps protect cells from damage, keeping the heart healthy and helping to prevent cancer. All tomatoes and tomato-based products, like tomato soup, tomato juice, and tomato sauce, contain lycopene. The body absorbs more lycopene when tomatoes are cooked and yet more in the presence of fat (e.g., cooking with oil or adding nuts to a tomato-based dish). Tomatoes also contain potassium, vitamin C, vitamin A, and beta-carotene.

Looking for more lycopene? Eat some watermelon!

Keep uncut watermelon at room temperature until it is fully ripe. Research shows, lycopene content increases during room temperature storage. Refrigerate watermelon once cut into pieces.

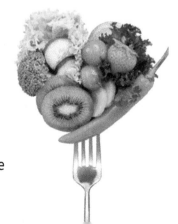

Homemade Tomato Sauce

Ingredients

- 1 TBSP garlic, minced
- 1 TBSP olive oil
- 1 (28 ounce) can crushed tomatoes*
- 1/2 cup tomato sauce*
- 2 TBSP + 1 TBSP tomato paste*
- 1 TBSP basil, dried
- 1 TBSP oregano, dried
- 1 TBSP parsley, dried
- ½ tsp sugar
- Salt and pepper to taste

*Use "no salt added" cans, if available.

Directions

1. In a medium sized pan, add the oil on medium heat.
2. Add the garlic and sauté for 2 – 3 minutes.
3. Add the crushed tomatoes, tomato sauce, 2 TBSP tomato paste, basil, oregano, parsley, sugar, salt, and pepper.
4. Stir and bring sauce to a boil.
5. Cover and simmer for 25 minutes. For a thicker consistency, add 1 TBSP tomato paste 15 minutes after the start of simmer.

Make it a Meal and Time it Well

Prepare the "*Turkey Meatballs*" pg. 58. Place them in the oven once the "Homemade Tomato Sauce" is ready to simmer. Start preparing the "*Sautéed Mushrooms*" pg. 16. Pick your favorite pasta and cook according to package.

Plate the pasta and meatballs. Pour the tomato sauce on top. Serve with a sprinkle of parmesan cheese and sautéed mushrooms on the side.

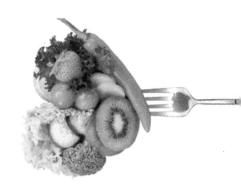

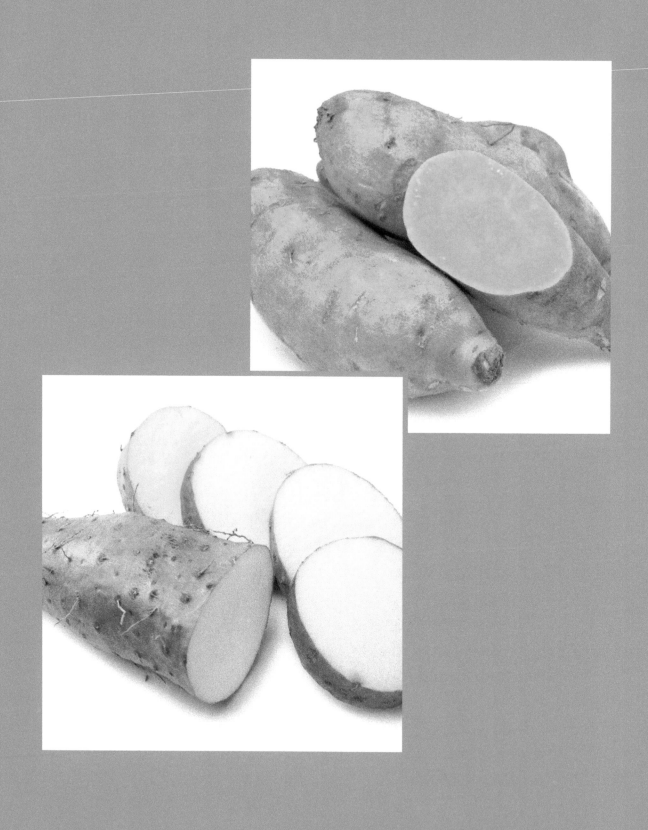

Do You Know The Differences Between Sweet Potatoes and Yams?

Sweet Potatoes	Yams
White, yellow, orange, purple, and red skin.	Brown, rough, hard to peel sometimes hairy skin.

Sweet and moist flesh
    White, orange, or purple flesh.
    White flesh sweet potatoes are not as sweet and moist as the darker skinned orange flesh sweet potatoes.
	Starchy and dry flesh
	    White, yellow, purple, or pink flesh.
	Usually not sweet.

Can often be found in local food stores.	Can be hard to find in local stores. Most often found in specialty or international food stores.
Grown in southern United States. Most crops grown in North Carolina.	Grown in tropical climates. Most crops grown in West Africa. Crops are also grown in South and Central America.

Sweet Potatoes Have:

- Beta carotene – The body changes beta carotene into vitamin A. Vitamin A helps keep the skin and eyes healthy and the immune system strong. Yams have a low amount of beta carotene.
- Fiber – helps with digestion and it helps to maintain fullness after eating a meal.
- Potassium – helps with fluid balance, muscle contractions, and nerve signals. Potassium also may help control your blood pressure.

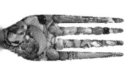

Say What?
Yams can grow to be 5 feet tall. Yams can be toxic if eaten raw. They must be cooked.

Garlicky Thyme Roasted Sweet Potatoes

Ingredients

- 2 large sweet potatoes, peeled and cut into 1-inch cubes
- 2 TBSP olive oil
- 1 TBSP garlic powder
- 2 tsp thyme, dried
- Salt and black pepper to taste

Directions

1. Preheat the oven to 425 degrees.
2. Mix the garlic powder and thyme in a small bowl.
3. In a medium sized bowl, toss the sweet potatoes in olive oil, then evenly sprinkle seasonings over them.
4. Lightly sprinkle with salt and pepper.
5. Place the potatoes on a baking sheet in a single layer.
6. Bake for 15 minutes, then turn the potatoes and cook for 10 -15 minutes more or until crispy.

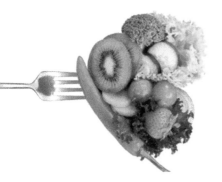

Oven Sweet Potato Fries

Ingredients

- 2 large sweet potatoes peeled and cut into ½ inch strips
- 2 TBSP olive oil
- 1 ½ tsp paprika
- 1 tsp onion powder
- 1 tsp garlic power
- ½ tsp chili powder

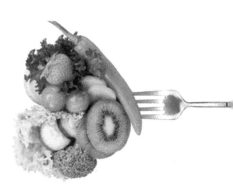

Directions

1. Preheat the oven to 425 degrees.
2. Mix the seasonings in a small bowl.
3. In a medium sized bowl, toss the sweet potatoes in olive oil then evenly sprinkle the seasonings over them.
4. Place the potatoes on a baking sheet in a single layer.
5. Bake 30 minutes or until golden brown.

> FACT: When your grocery store labels something a yam, more than likely, it's a sweet potato.

Sweet Potato Chips

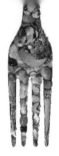

Ingredients

- 2 large sweet potatoes, peeled and sliced thinly
- 2 TBSP olive oil
- Salt to taste

Directions

1. Preheat the oven to 400 degrees.
2. In a medium sized bowl, toss together the olive oil and sweet potato slices. Sprinkle with salt.
3. Place the potatoes on a baking sheet in a single layer. Bake for 10 minutes, then turn the potatoes. Continue baking until tender and crispy on the edges, about 10 minutes more.

Note: The thinner you slice your potato, the more "chip" like the result will be. You may need to decrease time in the oven to prevent the potatoes from burning. The thinner the slices, the faster they will cook.

I love these sweet potato chips!

My mom submitted this recipe in a contest held at the day care I was attending at the time. The chips were selected to be on the lunch menu for a rotation.

Cinnamon Sweet Potato Chips

Ingredients

- 2 large sweet potatoes, peeled and sliced thinly
- 2 TBSP olive oil
- 2 tsp brown sugar
- 1 tsp ground cinnamon
- Salt to taste

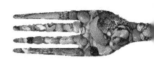

Directions

1. Preheat the oven to 400 degrees.
2. In a small bowl mix together the brown sugar and cinnamon.
3. In a medium sized bowl, toss together the olive oil and sweet potatoes.
4. Add the cinnamon mixture to the potatoes and toss until all coated. Sprinkle with salt.
5. Place the potatoes on a baking sheet in a single layer. Bake for 10 minutes, then turn the potatoes. Continue baking until tender and crispy on the edges, about 10 minutes more.

Try some YAMS

Add yams to the next stew, soup, or casserole prepared in the place of pasta, rice, or white potatoes. A purple fleshed yam, for sure, will be a topic of conversation at the dinner table.

Quick Mashed Yams:

Peel the skin of the yams then cut into similar-sized cubes. In a large pot, add enough water to cover the yams. Bring to a boil. Add yams and reduce heat to medium. Cook until fork tender, about 15 – 20 minutes. Drain then mash with a potato masher or fork. Add margarine, salt, and pepper to taste.

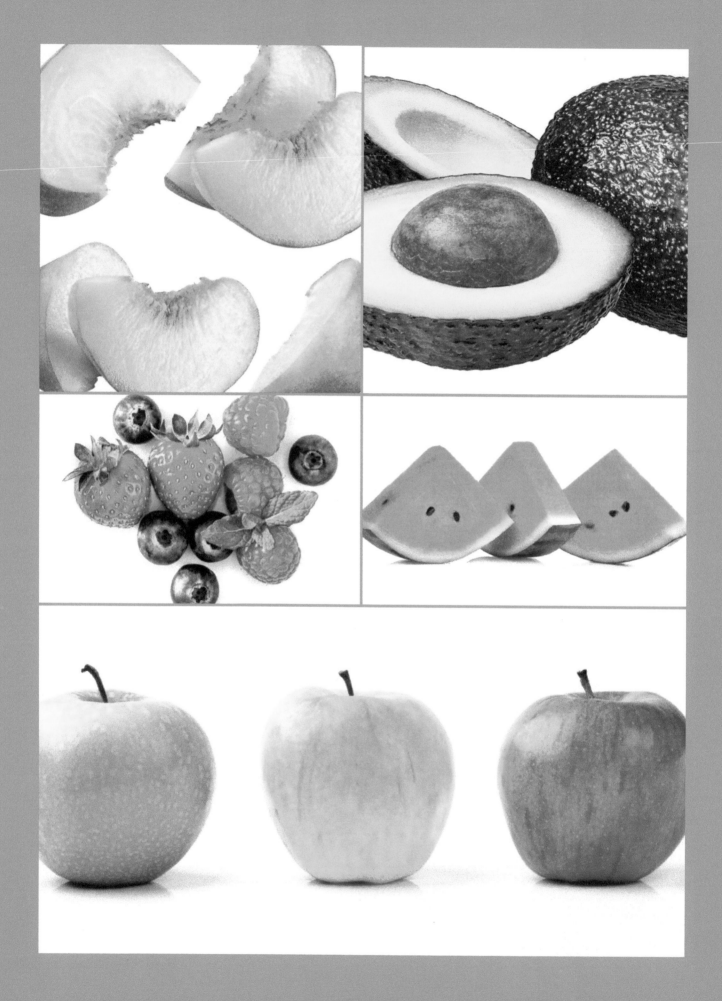

Why Fruits?

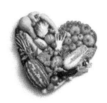

Low calories
Moderate to high carbohydrates
No dietary cholesterol
No fat (except avocado)
Low to high fiber
High in vitamins and minerals
Low sodium
Low protein
Low to high phytonutrients and antioxidants
Help maintain good health
Wide variety of flavors and textures

Fruits are rich in antioxidants. Antioxidants are substances that prevent damage to cells from free radicals. Too many free radicals in the body leads to diseases due to cell damage. Eating fruits are good for heart health and may help reduce the risk of infections and some forms of cancer. Increase your antioxidant intake by eating more nuts, seeds, beans, fruits, and vegetables.

Delicious Fruit Salad

This is easy to put together; keep it in the fridge and dish out in a bowl throughout the week.

You will need one cup of each: strawberries, oranges, blueberries, watermelon, cantaloupe, and honeydew.

- You may add 1 ½ to 2 cups of grapes.
- Slice the fruits to any size that pleases you.

In a medium to large sized bowl, combine the fruits together to create a healthful dish. Add some low-fat vanilla Greek yogurt to make it a filling snack. Serves 7.

Why Carbohydrates?

Carbohydrate is the body's main source of energy. The body needs carbohydrates like your car needs gas to run. Each fruit listed below has 15 grams of carbohydrate and 60 calories per serving.

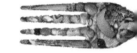

1 cup blackberries
¾ cup blueberries
1 cup cantaloupe diced
1 cup honeydew diced
1 cup raspberries
1 ¼ cup strawberries (whole)
1 ¼ cup watermelon diced

Other foods that contain carbohydrates include:

starchy vegetables, milk and yogurt, grains, beans, peas, lentils, and sugary foods and drinks.

> Which do you think are the least healthful?

Fresh Grilled Pineapple Wheels

Ingredients

- 1 pineapple, fresh and *ripe**
- 2 TBSP honey
- 1 TBSP lime juice, freshly squeezed
- 1 tsp olive oil
- 1 tsp chili powder

*Pick it Ripe!

Look for a pineapple with a fresh green stem and golden in color. The more yellow the pineapple looks, the riper it is.

Prepare Pineapple:

Cut off both ends of the pineapple. Stand the pineapple up. Run a knife along the outside of the fruit to shave off the tough outer skin. Cut the pineapple crosswise into ½ inch thick slices (about 6). Lay each slice flat. Using a knife, cut around the core (center) and discard. Place in a medium sized bowl.

Directions

1. In a small bowl, whisk together the honey, lime juice, oil, and chili powder.
2. Pour mixture over the pineapple. Make sure each slice is well coated. Place in the refrigerator for about 15 minutes.
3. Meanwhile, heat grill to medium to high heat. Lightly oil the grill rack.
4. Put pineapple slices on the grill in a single layer.
5. Cook for 5 minutes on each side or until golden brown and tender. Serves 6.

No Grill?

Broil pineapple in the oven for 3-4 minutes on each side.

Serve as a side with pork, chicken, or salmon.

Note: Canned pineapple in natural juice may be used if fresh pineapples are not available.

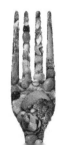

Why Avocados?

One-third of a medium avocado has 80 calories and around 20 vitamins, minerals, and phytonutrients, making it a heart-healthy fruit. Most of the fats in the diet should be unsaturated, heart-healthy monounsaturated, or polyunsaturated. More than 75 percent of the fat in avocados is monounsaturated.

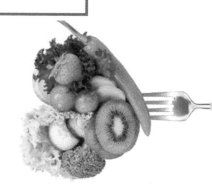

Note: Avocados do not have sodium, sugar, nor do they have dietary cholesterol, as they are a plant food.

Avocado Garlic Spread

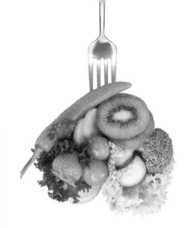

Ingredients

- 2 avocados, soft and ripe
- 2 TBSP garlic, minced
- 1/2 tsp lemon juice
- Salt to taste

Try with "Homemade Pita Chips" pg. 51.

Directions

1. Cut each avocado lengthwise around the seed.
2. Rotate the halves to separate.
3. Using a spoon, remove the seed and scoop the avocado into a bowl.
4. Mash the avocado.
5. Press the garlic into the avocado, add lemon juice, and salt. Mix well.

You can put this spread on bread, bagels, or crackers. It makes a great dip for raw carrots, cucumbers, broccoli, and sweet peppers. It's amazing eaten from a big spoon, too!

Keep unused spread in the refrigerator. To help prevent browning, sprinkle a little lemon juice on top and press a piece of plastic wrap directly against the spread in a sealed container.

"This is my new mayonnaise."

—Debra A. Conyers, BSN, RN, B.Sc.,
Food Science and Nutrition

Go A Little Nuts Over NUTS

Research shows eating a variety of nuts and nut butters can decrease the risk of heart disease and help improve blood pressure.

Good choices are:

- almonds
- hazelnuts
- peanuts*
- pecans
- pistachios
- walnuts

*FACT: Peanuts are legumes but are often grouped with nuts. Legumes are the edible seeds enclosed in pods. Peanuts are in the same family as beans, peas, and lentils.

Nuts provide:

- vitamins
  - E
  - folate
- minerals
  - calcium
  - magnesium
  - potassium
- antioxidants
- unsaturated fats
- protein
- fiber

"A handful, not a can-full" is all you need to get the benefits!

Try to buy unsalted nuts OR mix salted with unsalted to make your handful.

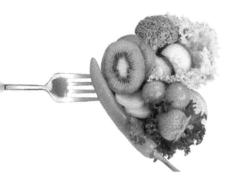

Avoid chocolate and sugar-coated nuts.

Sweet Gala Apple Medley

Ingredients

- 2 medium gala apples, cut in bite size cubes
- ¼ cup red onion, chopped
- 1/3 cup celery, chopped
- ¼ cup walnuts, chopped (optional)
- 1 cup can black beans, rinsed and drained
- 2 TBSP apple cider vinegar
- 2 tsp honey
- 2 tsp Dijon mustard

Directions

1. Combine the apples, onions, celery, nuts, and black beans in a bowl.
2. In another bowl mix the vinegar, honey, and mustard.
3. Pour over the apple mixture and stir gently to coat.
4. Refrigerate for at least 1 hour or overnight.

Note: You can replace gala apples with your favorite sweet apple. Other sweet apples include red delicious, honeycrisp, and fuji.

> Walnuts are an excellent source of omega-3 fatty acids. Omega-3 fatty acids help to prevent heart disease and reduce inflammation.

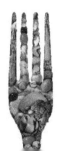

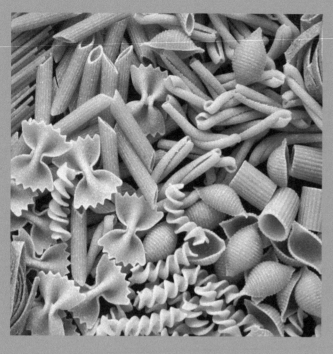

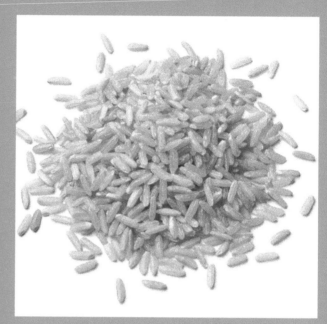

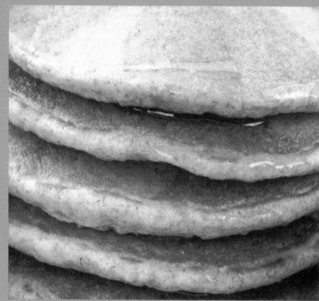

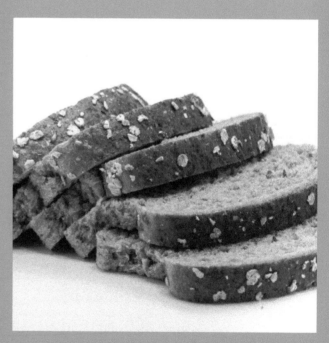

Why Whole Grains?

Whole Grains vs. Refined Grains

- Whole grains contain the entire grain kernel—the bran, germ, and endosperm (very nutritious).
- Refined grains have been milled, a process that removes the bran and germ (not as nutritious).

Whole Grains Are

- High in carbohydrates which provide energy
- Low in fat
- Beneficial for digestive health
- High in folate which can help repair tissue
- Good source of B-vitamins, iron, magnesium, and selenium
- High in fiber which helps reduce heart disease

Make sure you don't rely on color or texture of your grain. Be sure "whole" is the first word on the ingredient list. Examples of whole grains are brown rice, whole wheat bread, oatmeal, and popcorn.

More about whole grains

Foods labeled with the words below are usually *not* whole grain products:

multi-grain	*stone-ground*
100% wheat	*cracked wheat*
seven-grain	*bran*

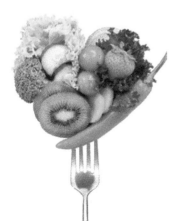

Weekend Pancakes

Ingredients

Dry Ingredients:
- 1 cup all-purpose flour
- ½ cup whole wheat flour
- 1 TBSP baking powder
- 1 TBSP sugar
- ½ tsp salt

Wet Ingredients:
- 1 cup milk
- 2 TBSP canola oil
- 1 egg (or 2 egg whites)
- 1 tsp vanilla extract

Directions

1. In a medium sized bowl, combine the dry ingredients.
2. In another bowl, whisk together the wet ingredients.
3. Slowly fold the liquid into the dry ingredients. Stir until a thick, smooth consistency. It's okay to have a few lumps. If the batter is too thick, (does not pour easily from a spoon), stir in 1-2 TBSP milk until desired consistency is met.
4. Heat a griddle or non-stick pan on low to medium heat. Lightly grease the pan. Slowly pour ¼ cup of batter for each pancake into the pan until round.
5. When the pan side is golden and bubbles appear on surface, flip the pancakes, and cook until golden brown. Repeat steps with remaining batter.

Serve with honey, maple syrup or "Berrylicious Topping" on pg. 45.

Note: To increase the fiber in this recipe, you can replace the all-purpose flour with whole wheat flour which may make the batter a little thicker. Add 1-2 TBSP of milk to your batter until desired consistency is met.

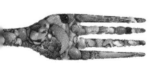

Berrylicious Topping

Ingredients

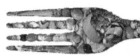

- 3 cups berries, fresh or frozen (strawberries, blackberries, blueberries, raspberries)
- 3 TBSP sugar
- 2 TBSP water

Directions

1. In a saucepan, combine the berries, sugar, and water.
2. Bring to a boil and cook for 1 minute. Stir the mixture to keep it from burning and sticking to the pan.
3. Reduce heat and simmer for about 15 minutes or until a thick consistency.

Use as a topping for pancakes or waffles.

Note: If using large berries, cut into bite size pieces.

Why Fiber?

Fiber is a carbohydrate found in plant foods such as fruits, vegetables, beans, nuts, and whole grains. The body cannot break down or absorb fiber therefore has NO CALORIES. Research shows many benefits to eating foods with fiber, such as:

- Promotes regular bowel movements, keeping digestive system healthy
- Lowers the risk for cancer
- Helps with weight control, keeping you satisfied after eating a meal
- Helps control blood sugar, therefore, it's good for people with diabetes
- Lower LDL levels (bad cholesterol), making it good for the heart

Why Pumpkin?

Pumpkin has many nutrients. It is rich in beta-carotene which turns to vitamin A in the body. Pumpkin has vitamin C, too. Both vitamins A and C can help boost the immune system. Fiber, potassium, and iron are three additional nutrients found in pumpkin.

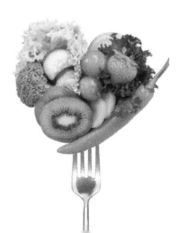

Jada's Pumpkin Applesauce Muffins

Ingredients

Wet ingredients:

- 2 eggs
- 1 cup canned pumpkin
- ¼ cup canola oil
- ½ cup applesauce

Dry ingredients:

- ½ cup sugar
- ½ cup light brown sugar
- 1¾ cup all-purpose flour
- 2 ½ tsp pumpkin pie spice
- 1 tsp baking soda
- ½ tsp salt

Directions

1. Preheat the oven to 375 degrees. Line two standard muffin tins with paper liners and set aside (12 muffins total).
2. In a large bowl, whisk together the wet ingredients.
3. In a separate bowl, stir together the dry ingredients.
4. Add the dry ingredients to the wet ingredients and mix until just combined (do not overmix or the muffins may be dense and kind of heavy).
5. Divide the batter evenly among the prepared muffin tins, filling the cups about ⅔ full.
6. Bake for 20 minutes until the top of the muffins spring back to the touch and/or a toothpick inserted in the center of a muffin comes out clean or with a few moist crumbs attached.
7. Remove the muffins from the tin to let them cool.

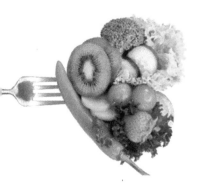

To increase the fiber in this recipe, replace ½ cup of the all-purpose flour with whole wheat flour:

- 1 ¼ cup all-purpose flour plus ½ cup whole wheat flour

Why Not Buttermilk?

Buttermilk is high in sodium. One cup can equal:

464 mg sodium   fat-free or low-fat buttermilk

256 mg sodium   2% or whole buttermilk

Note: Though 2% and whole buttermilk is lower in sodium, keep in mind they are higher in the fat that is not good for the heart.

To lower the sodium in any recipe that calls for buttermilk, mix 1 cup of milk and 1 TBSP of lemon juice or white vinegar. Remember to let it set at room temperature for 5-10 minutes before using.

> Surprisingly, buttermilk does not contain butter. Traditional buttermilk is the liquid leftover after milk has been churned into butter.

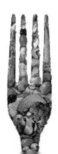

No Buttermilk Cornbread

Ingredients

Dry ingredients:

- 1 cup all-purpose flour
- ¾ cup yellow cornmeal
- 2 tsp baking powder
- ½ tsp salt
- 2 TBSP sugar

Wet ingredients:

- 1 cup + ¼ cup milk
- 1 TBSP white vinegar (or lemon juice)
- 1 egg
- 1/3 cup canola oil

Directions

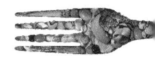

1. Preheat the oven to 400 degrees.
2. Gently mix 1 cup milk and the white vinegar. Let the mixture sit for at least 5 – 10 minutes. It should begin to slightly thicken and curdle (this is a replacement for buttermilk).
3. Mix the dry ingredients.
4. In another bowl, beat the egg then add oil and both milks.
5. Mix well.
6. Add the liquid to the flour mixture. Mix just until moistened.
7. Put the mixture into a greased 8-inch square baking pan.
8. Bake for 30 – 35 minutes.

Spread some margarine on top while hot out of the oven!

What About the Other Milk?

Milk, along with cheese and yogurt, is a good source of calcium. Calcium is important for bone health, heart and muscle function, and blood clotting. Vitamin D is needed to absorb calcium in the body.

Other sources of calcium include dark, leafy greens, soybeans, and fortified juices and cereals.

> Spinach is one of many dark, leafy greens that contains calcium. However, spinach is high in the compound, oxalate, that binds to calcium and reduces its absorption.

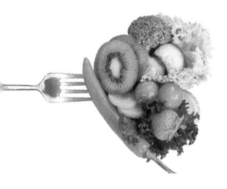

FACT: 99% of all calcium in the body is stored in the bones.

Homemade Pita Chips

Ingredients

- 2 ½ whole pitas
- 2 TBSP olive oil
- 1 tsp onion powder
- 1 ½ tsp garlic powder
- 1 tsp basil, dried
- Salt to taste

Enjoy with "Avocado Garlic Spread" pg. 39, hummus, bean dip, or salsa for a healthful good tasting snack.

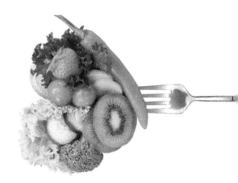

Directions

1. Preheat the oven to 375 degrees.
2. Using a pizza cutter, cut each pita into 8 triangles.
3. Pita pieces will easily split at the seams to make two pieces.
4. Arrange the pita pieces in a single layer on a baking sheet.
5. Mix in a small bowl the oil, onion powder, garlic powder, basil, and salt.
6. Brush one side of each pita piece with the oil mixture. Seasonings will settle at the bottom of the bowl, so stir the mixture with the brush as you are coating each piece.
7. Bake for 6 - 8 minutes.

Let cool. Store leftovers in an airtight container up to 2 days.

Note: Use whole wheat pitas to increase fiber and other nutrients.

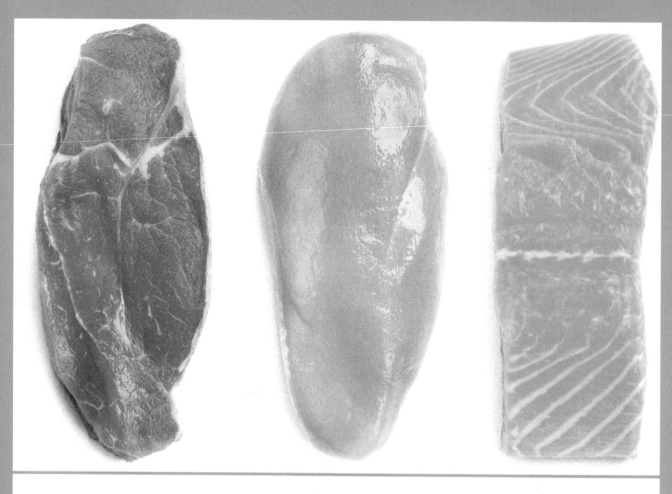

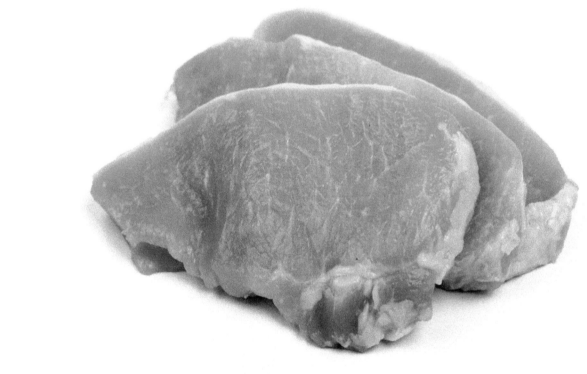

Cholesterol is...

...a fatty substance found in the blood. It is used by the body to make hormones and build cells. The liver makes cholesterol, but we also get it from animal foods such as meat, butter, eggs, cheese, and milk. When we eat too much fat, especially saturated fat, it causes the liver to make too much cholesterol, which is not good for the heart.

To reduce dietary cholesterol, try to limit how much red meat you eat. Select turkey, chicken, and fish more often. Drink fat-free or 1% milk and eat low-fat yogurt. Remember moderation when you eat butter, eggs, and cheese. Dietary cholesterol is only found in animal foods, never plant foods.

More About Milk

One cup equals:

	Total Fat Grams	Saturated Fat Grams
Whole Milk	8	5
Low-fat milk	3	1.5

Got Lactose Intolerance?

Lactose intolerance is when the body cannot break down the carbohydrate lactose. Lactase is an enzyme needed to break down lactose. If the body does not make enough lactase, this will cause bloating, stomach cramps and/or diarrhea. Try lactose free milk or milk alternatives: rice milk, soy milk, almond and other nut milk options.

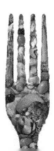

Skillet Salmon

Ingredients

- 4 (4-ounce) salmon filets, 1 inch thick
- 2 TBSP olive oil
- Salt and black pepper to taste

Directions

1. Remove the salmon from the refrigerator and let stand at room temperature for 10 minutes.
2. Meanwhile, heat the oil in skillet over medium heat.
3. Lightly sprinkle the salmon with salt and pepper.
4. Increase heat to medium high. Place the salmon, skin side UP, in the skillet.
5. Cook until golden brown on 1 side, about 4 minutes. Turn the salmon over and cook until it feels firm to the touch and the skin is crisp, about 2 - 3 minutes more.

> Salmon is a fatty fish with a rich content of protein and omega-3 fatty acids. Omega-3 fatty acids help to prevent heart disease and reduce inflammation.

Why room temperature?

Salmon, like most fish, does not take long to cook. Once your fish is completely thawed in the refrigerator, let it warm up to room temperature before cooking (about 10 minutes). The colder the fish is before cooking, the more likely you are to overcook the outside of the fish before the inside is finished.

Lemon Herb Salmon

Ingredients

- 4 (4-ounce) salmon filets, 1 inch thick
- 1 ½ TBSP olive oil
- Zest* and juice of 1 small lemon
- 1 TBSP garlic, minced
- 1 tsp dried rosemary
- 1 tsp dried thyme
- ¼ tsp black pepper

*Scrape the outer peel of the lemon.

Directions

1. Preheat the oven to 350 degrees.
2. Remove the salmon from the refrigerator and let stand at room temperature for 10 minutes.
3. In a small bowl, whisk together all the ingredients except the salmon.
4. Skin side DOWN, place the salmon in a greased baking dish and spoon lemon mixture evenly on each piece of salmon. Gently rub to coat.
5. Bake the salmon for 15-20 minutes, until it is almost completely cooked through at the thickest part. The cooking time will vary based on the thickness of the salmon.

Note: When the salmon flakes easily with a fork, it is ready.

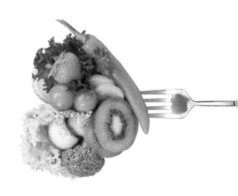

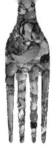

Looking for just salmon and lemon?

Follow steps 1, 2, and 5 under Lemon Herb Salmon. Adjust Steps 3 and 4 to the following:

Step 3: Skin side DOWN, place the salmon in a greased baking dish and drizzle with oil and a little honey (honey, optional). Lightly sprinkle with salt and pepper.

Step 4: Cut a lemon in half. Squeeze lemon juice evenly on the pieces of salmon.

> Note: In addition to salmon, mackerel, herring, lake trout, sardines, and albacore tuna are also fatty fish rich in omega-3 fatty acids.

Additionally, walnuts are good sources of omega-3 fatty acids.

Why Iron?

Iron is needed to carry oxygen to the lungs, muscles, and all parts of the body. Iron also helps with brain function and helps keep the immune system strong. Iron is found in both animal and plant foods. Sources of both are found below.

Animal sources:
- Lean beef and pork
- Chicken and turkey
- Fish and other seafood

> *Tofu is a plant-based protein that is made from curdling soymilk and forming it into a solid block.

Plant sources:
- Beans and lentils
- Leafy green vegetables like spinach and kale
- Whole grains and fortified breads and cereals
- Tofu*

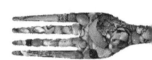

The body absorbs the iron from animal sources more easily than from plant foods. Combining foods rich in vitamin C in the same meal with high iron foods, will improve the absorption of the iron.

Vitamin C rich foods:

Brussel sprouts, broccoli, cabbage, cauliflower, green and red bell peppers, potatoes, spinach, tomatoes, strawberries, and citrus fruits like pineapples, oranges, lemons, limes, and grapefruits.

Try some of these iron rich plant foods and vitamin C combinations:

Oatmeal + Strawberries
Kale + Lemon
Lentils + Tomatoes
Beans + Red Peppers
Pinto Beans + Cabbage

(*"Lemony Kale Spaghetti"* pg. 23)
(*"Herb Tomato & Cucumber Medley"* pg. 10)
(*"Three Bean Salad"* pg. 21)
(*"Mama's Beans"* pg. 5 and *"Grandma's Cabbage"* pg. 7)

Note: Some foods and beverages may cause the body to absorb less iron when eaten close together. If you have low iron, a registered dietitian (RD) or registered dietitian nutritionist (RDN) will help you develop an eating plan that's right for you.

Turkey Meat Balls

Ingredients

- 1-pound ground turkey
- 1 egg
- ¼ cup parmesan cheese
- ¾ cup Italian style breadcrumbs
- 1 ½ TBSP Italian seasoning, salt free

Directions

1. Preheat the oven to 350 degrees.
2. Combine all ingredients and form them into balls (the size of ping pong balls).
3. Bake for 20-25 minutes or until done.

These are perfect with "Homemade Tomato Sauce" pg. 27.

In a hurry?
Add your favorite jar of tomato sauce. Be cautious, some brands are higher in sodium than others.

Pork Loin Sauteed with Peaches

Ingredients

- 1 TBSP + 1 tsp olive oil
- 1-pound fresh pork loin cut in cubes
- Salt and black pepper to taste
- ¼ cup onions, chopped
- 1 tsp dried thyme
- 2 peaches cut into wedges
- ½ cup apple cider vinegar
- ½ cup low sodium chicken broth
- 2 tsp honey

Directions

1. Heat 1 TBSP oil in a pan on medium heat. Season the cubed pork with salt and pepper and cook until done. Remove the pork from the pan and set aside.
2. Add the remaining oil, onions, thyme, and peaches to the pan, cook for two minutes.
3. Stir in the vinegar and bring to a boil. Cook until reduced to 1/3 cup, about 2 minutes.
4. Stir in the broth and honey, bring back to a boil. Cook until reduced to 1/3 cup, about 2 minutes.
5. Remove from heat. Add the pork, mix, and enjoy on top of your favorite whole grain. My favorite whole grain is brown rice.

Note: You can use 1 – 15 oz can of peaches, drained and rinsed in place of fresh peaches.

Mushroomed Burgers

Ingredients

- 1-pound lean ground beef (85% fat free)
- 2 TBSP Worcestershire sauce
- ¾ cup mushrooms, chopped
- 2 TBSP garlic, minced
- Salt and black pepper to taste
- 1 egg, beaten
- ¼ cup Italian style breadcrumbs

Directions

1. Preheat the oven to 350 degrees.
2. Mix all the ingredients together in a bowl.
3. Shape into four patties.
4. Place the patties on a greased baking sheet.
5. Bake until done as desired (well done is about 20 – 25 minutes).

> Serve with spinach or lettuce leaves, sliced tomatoes, and onions on a toasted bun.

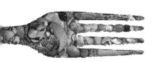

Want more mushrooms?
Top burgers with "Sauted Mushrooms" pg. 16.

Apricot Chicken

Ingredients

- 1 TBSP olive oil
- 1 ½ pounds boneless, skinless chicken thighs
- Salt and black pepper to taste
- 1 cup low sodium chicken broth
- Zest and juice of 1 small lemon
- 1 ½ TBSP Dijon mustard
- 1 TBSP garlic, minced
- 1 tsp dried thyme
- ¾ cup sliced onion
- ¾ cup dried apricots, cut in half

Directions

1. Sear the chicken (heat oil over medium high heat in a large pan. Season the chicken with salt and pepper and brown for about 2 ½ minutes on each side).
2. Meanwhile, in a small bowl, mix the broth, lemon zest and juice, mustard, garlic, and thyme. Whisk until blended well.
3. Add the broth mixture, onions, and apricots to the chicken and bring to a boil for less than 10 seconds.
4. Reduce heat, cover, and simmer for 25 – 30 minutes or until the chicken is fully cooked.

Serve on top of brown rice or your favorite whole grain.

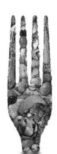

Registered Dietitian

A registered dietitian or registered dietitian nutritionist can help you manage medical conditions like prediabetes, diabetes, high blood pressure, high cholesterol, and heart disease. A RD or RDN will partner with you to create an eating plan that is safe, realistic, and has the nutrients needed to manage your condition. Visit eatright.org to locate a RD or RDN near you.

A registered dietitian who specializes in diabetes is a certified diabetes care education specialists (CDCES). Visit diabeteseducator.org to locate a CDCES near you.

> Note: All registered dietitians are nutritionists, but not all nutritionists are registered dietitians.

For more healthful recipes and nutrition information, please visit:

Academy of Nutrition and Dietetics
eatright.org

American Diabetes Association
diabetes.org

American Heart Association
heart.org

United States Department of Agriculture
myplate.gov

Resources

Academy of Nutrition and Dietetics
eatright.org

International Food Information
Council
foodinsight.org

American Diabetes Association
diabetes.org

NC Sweet Potatoes
ncsweetpotatoes.com

American Egg Board
aeb.org

US Dry Bean Council
usdrybeans.com

American Heart Association
heart.org

US Food and Drug Administration
fda.gov

American Institute for Cancer
Research
aicr.org

United States Department of
Agriculture
USDA.org
National Agricultural Library
FoodData Central
myplate.gov

California Avocados
californiaavocado.com

Alphabetical List of Recipes

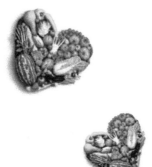

Index

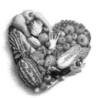

About the Author

Jada Johnson is currently in the 12th grade and stays on the honor roll. During her first 17 years of life, she has accomplished many things:

1. Girl Scout currently in her 10th year of membership. She is an Ambassador and a proud 2020 recipient of the Girl Scout Gold Award, the highest award a girl scout can achieve.
2. Numerous awards and recognitions playing the cello.
3. Earned her second degree blackbelt in karate.
4. Member of the Diamonds in the Rough step team.
5. Most recent achievement, author, and publisher of,

Food Is Medicine
Nutritious and Delicious Recipes from my home shared with you

Jada's love for cooking comes from her dad. Her knowledge of nutrition comes from her mom.

Jada understands and knows the importance of volunteerism, helping others, and giving back to the community. Her choice of a career in healthcare is her next step.

The Meaning of Jada's R.O.A.R.

The company Jada's R.O.A.R., LLC was created because I want to encourage girls and women of all ages to be heard. Make sure your opinion is known to others. If you have an idea, then say it! This may be your only shot to do so. Always make sure you voice your opinion respectfully; as a result, your peers will show respect towards you. Ladies, stay confident and courageous in new adventures, and know we can achieve so much if all of us would R.O.A.R...

Reach Out And Rule!